"FOOD POLITRICKS

ARE YOU EATING YOURSELF TO

DEATH?™ "

Conrad J. Cornelius

This book is livicated to my father, Mr. Conrad I. Cornelius, a.k.a. C.I.C. You are a true leader and a real inspiration. The seeds that you planted, have now grown into trees; bearing much fruits in our season. The lessons that you have taught us will be remembered by our children's children...

Be reminded that the journey has only just started. I pray that you continue in health, strength, and prosperity. Thank you so very much.

Table of Contents

Introduction

The purpose of this book is to help us to really question our own eating habits. Is what we eat really that important? How important are our food choices? How does it affect our health and overall life span in general? Are we really eating ourselves to an early grave? Should we even care?

It is becoming more and more evident that a significant amount of us are paying no real attention to the foods that we eat. On the other hand, a rising number of us are paying greater attention as to what we feast on and the effect on our health. We become living examples that there is a serious relationship between the food we eat and our overall health. Just ask David Wolfe. He would tell you.

The story goes on. In my eleven (11) years of experience as the founder of Natural Livity Inc. (a Vegan Café` franchise project), a Personal Chef, and a Holistic Health Care Consultant; I have seen solid evidence to support this reality. The foods that we eat does indeed affect our health and wellness. There is also a definite relationship between what we eat and how we think, function, and live.

I have listened to arguments from both sides of the fence, and the food debate can go on forever. I myself have been on both sides of the fence since I was not always a vegan. In my own analysis, I must admit that there are many benefits eating from Mother Nature's menu. Such great benefits, that I am always very thankful to the Creator for all these life giving gifts. I found it important to ask myself the question. It was even more important for me to make changes to the diet that I was fed growing up. Life is here for all of us in abundance. It is one of Nature's joys as our Mother to feed us the very best.

This is what I have grown to believe and know to be true! What do you believe?

Some people say that as long as you are alive, the day of death is sure. Does that give us the right to eat everything that we can possibly get our teeth on? This is the basic environment that the majority of us grow up in as far as tips towards general nutrition. It was basically catch, kill, cook, and eat (with the exception of insects and bugs etc)! Who started that anyway? Crabs, iguanas, agoutis, and manikou are all ok to eat some say. At one time mountain chicken, (a frog) was claimed to be the national dish on my island of Dominica. As strange that this may sound, it is the truth. All too often the tragic results of eating this way on a long term are sickness, disease, and medical drugs. The end of this journey is usually death. Shouldn't we be considering the consequences?

This book is an attempt to help us open up and question our own minds as to food choices we make today. It also serves to help us to question some of the recipes that were handed down to us from tradition, as it relates to food and nutritional health. Many of us have lost loved ones and we know we can't bring them back. Life is an experience and the opportunity to learn from the mistakes of others, can add years of health and happiness to our own lives and the lives of those we presently love so much. Life was created for the living. We are aware that we cannot change the past, but we sure can use the past to influence a much greater future.

You may find some repetition within these pages. This is willful and done for emphasis. Get this message clear. Our lives and that of our children and love ones are at stake here. If we don't question the choices we make now, we are most likely to fall victim to the mistakes of those who have already passed on. The causes of the majority of Chronic Non Communicable Diseases (CNCDs) like diabetes, high blood pressure, obesity, cancers, and strokes, etc; have been directly linked to poor food choices, bad eating habits, and lack of exercise.

No one should have to die because they were uninformed or wrongly educated about the food choices to make at meal time. No one! Especially when loving Mother Nature continues to grow such a huge variety of much healthier options for us. Now I am asking you this question. Are you really eating yourself to death? The topic of **"Food Politricks"** continues to investigate this all important issue. Know yourself and comprehend. Know your worth!

.

The Gift of Life

Life is a very precious gift! A treasure like no other, we have to admit. To be able to experience so many wonders, cannot be compared to career, sports, or hobbies put together. Life gives us everything we can possible think of. I have a challenge for you. Name me one thing that Mother Earth is without? While you are at it, do take some time to breathe. Inhale, exhale, and give thanks for life. Without this breath of life, you could never be alive to read this. Correct or natural Food sustains this life force. Nature provides all the nutrients, minerals, vitamins, and other trace elements in a way that only Nature can provide. All our wants and needs are supplied. As the ALL Wise and Knowing One said; *'be close to me and I will be close to you... you shall not want'.*

Why are so many of us, even the richest and most educated, victims of unwanted sickness, disease, and death? Could it be because of something so simple as incorrect food choices and bad eating habits? It becomes very strange when you truly analyze the root cause of the many Chronic Non Communicable Diseases (CNCD's) and relative discomforts currently plaguing the peoples of the world. The World Health Organization has admitted that over consumption of processed and unnatural foods are claiming the lives of millions. It is time to stop this misery. Much too many of our dearly beloved have already passed on. Now our children - who are our future - are much too precious to allow ourselves as parents and guardians, to teach them to adopt this self-destructive "lifestyle!"

Some of the major diseases are diabetes, obesity, high blood pressure, lack of energy (fatigue), heart conditions, and strokes etc. When we take a closer look into the causes of these diseases, we will see that all these have been directly linked in some form or another to poor nutrition and lack of exercise. Wrong food choices and bad eating habits are claiming the lives of millions of us every year.

According to Henry G. Bieler, M.D. in his tremendous work as the author of *"Food is Your Best Medicine"*; he states, *'As a practicing physician for over fifty years, I have reached three basic conclusions as to the cause and cure of disease... The first is that the primary cause of disease is not germs. Rather, I believe that disease is caused by a toxemia which results in cellular impairment and breakdown, thus paving the way for the multiplication and onslaught of germs. My second conclusion is that in almost all cases, the use of drugs in treating patients is harmful. Drugs often cause serious side effects, and sometimes even create new diseases. ...The physician is indeed rare who can be completely aware of the potential danger from the side effects of all of these drugs. My third conclusion is that disease can be cured through the proper use of correct foods...'*

It is becoming evident that the root of the problem is being dished out at the breakfast tables (for those who even have time to eat breakfast), at the lunch counters, and on the dinner plates. In addition to these three square meals, most of us have an addiction to processed snacks and other forms of "junk" food and artificial drinks. These are usually over-packed with salt, unsaturated fats, dangerous additives, artificial sugars, and chemical preservatives.

The human body is one of the most amazing mechanisms ever created! Thus, we should learn to value and take the utmost care of ourselves. We only have one body vehicle. It would be very sad to know that we are the ones most responsible for our own destruction. The foods we eat; what we eat, when we eat, and why we eat, are responsible for our health. The Creator has provided such wide variety of natural food, of every taste and delight, to sustain us in perfect health – mind, body, and soul — that we lack nothing.

Yet the majority of us these days will say no to a grapefruit or a glass of pure orange juice, but say yes to a soft drink/soda. Most would pass up on a cup of herbal tea for a glass of cow's milk. A young lady recently said to me "I don't drink grass. No, I don't drink bush". It gets worse at lunch time where any kind of meat, salt, oil, and white sugar become the special order of the day. Some wonder at the end of the day why do they feel so tired? The reason is this. Most of these processed foods contain little to no nutritional value. They actually tend to take from the body instead of feeding the cells with life giving energy. The stomach is filled yes, but the cells stay hungry.

Food is the staff of life. Preparing and cooking meals is a natural form of therapy. With true knowledge and your choice of natural ingredients, gourmet meals can be created in little time. Part of the issue is that the demands of society leave us with so little free time. Or should I say most of our time is spent away from our own kitchens. Now food and where to eat becomes a headache. Many of us would like to maintain a healthy lifestyle. We want to feel energetic and vibrant. We need to begin to understand that it starts with what we eat. Natural Livity Inc. is here to help fill this need.

Take a car for example. You may have the best car. If you do not put sufficient water into the radiator, and do not change your oil and filters regularly enough, and if you use the lowest grade of gasoline; in a short time you are going to experience difficulties with this car.

Unfortunately, this is the situation with so many of us. The Almighty Creator has given us such an amazing gift. We should feed our cells the best possible nutrients. Instead we feed on the worse possible ingredients and still expect to live a long joyful life. The reality of the situation is that many of us take better care of our cars and trucks than we take care of ourselves.

I think it is time that we (I say we because I am right in this with you) gain a better understanding of how the body really works. How does it react to the different foods that we eat? It is now an accepted joke to be feeling sleepy after lunch. In the world of wiser choices and proper nutrition, there is no need for that droopy feeling. Companies would see an increase in productivity and profits if they were to encourage their employees to eat from a healthier menu at lunch time. This current fast food trend will continue to result in more sick days and a higher health care bill. Company owners should look into this.

The lunch plate is usually filled with starch, favorite animal body parts, fats and oils, table salt (inorganic sodium chloride) and a sprinkle of vegetables as a salad (if any). There is also the ever present soft drink or soda which is packed with large amounts of artificial colorings and sweeteners. All this is eaten within ten to fifteen minutes, and then we are off to work again. Those of us who have active jobs stand a better chance than those who have office jobs. Sitting alert after lunch in that office, cubicle, or at those desks is usually the hardest part of the job. A dangerous habit forms. And without proper exercise, this commonly spells the road to fatigue, obesity, her friends and followers.

The body now has to work extra to balance off this

rush of foreign substances. This balancing process requires more energy than the meal we just ate can provide. Instead of gaining energy, we lose energy and this tired and sleepy feeling kicks in. The energy needed to be active is being used up to break down all this "food" that was eaten for lunch. Without sufficient movement and exercise, anyone subjected to this routine will eventually find themselves starting to show skin disorders and signs of obesity. Naturally a host of other things are going wrong on the inside as well. A young man may find himself losing his hair (baldness), growing pot bellies, and having complications like impotence. In addition to obesity, women usually suffer from irregular menstrual cycles, fibroids, acne, and headaches, etc.

There are many diseases associated with a destructive eating cycle. Truthfully speaking, there is nothing really mysterious about most of the things that happen to us and around us. The difficulty is that most of us cannot find the time to study what is truly going on. Others have no interest in getting to the root of things. Most of us simply go with the flow. It does not matter if this flow is in keeping with who we are or who we would like to be. The cliché "shit in shit out" holds very true today more than ever. Think of it like this "we are what we eat!" Think about it.

This experience called life is much too important to neglect the natural laws that have been governing the entire universe from since creation was given birth, and lunch time began. There are a variety of fruits, vegetables, herbs, beans, and other natural forms of food which can be eaten naturally or prepared in a variety of recipes which could satisfy every taste and need known to man. For some reason or another, do we no longer find them tasty and satisfying? Or do we simply need correct education and healthier menu options? The story goes on.

Why aren't we exposed to a more natural menu? Why would most children turn up their face at the sight of a carrot? And why would these same children cry long tears if we say no to that lollipop or corn curls they wanted? Why is there this apparent conditioning to quickly accept such things that would damage our structure? Why do we seem to reject those things which would add such benefits to our life? It is amazing how many questions studying the relationship between our health and the food that we eat could bring about. As complicated as it may seem, as complicated as it may sound, it is worth taking a good look into. Lack of health knowledge and awareness can cost you your life! How is that for complication?

Making Healthier Choices

We have a choice in designing our life and future. It would be for the improvement of humanity if we all would take a closer look into the very necessary process we know as Eating. Most of us don't pay much attention to that which our life depends on. Many are clueless as to what is happening in the environment. Most of us just go along our merry way, following the crowd, doing what we must to survive. When we begin to suffer, there are experts to whom we are referred. These experts advise us at very high costs as to what we must do. Our spending continues because these experts usually send us on to the drug stores and pharmacies. These pharmaceutical companies make billions of dollars a year selling drugs. Most of us are almost desperate to get relief from the dis-ease and discomfort that we experience, that we buy and use these drugs.

Grand Ma always said that "Prevention is Better than Cure!" Have you ever analyzed the true meaning of this proverb? The moral of the story is that it is better to prevent an injury than to find the solution necessary to nurse the wound. For example, keep your car in proper condition. Service regularly and check that there is sufficient water and oil for proper performance. What happens? Ok. Now pay no good attention to the car and allow this car to breakdown? What happens?

The money that you spend to fix the car would be much more that the costs of the regular checks. You would now have to buy auto parts, pay the mechanic to restore this car to good working condition, and spend time without the use of your car. Getting to and from work now becomes so much more difficult. It may seem like a hassle to go through with these regular visits to the auto care shop. But in the long run these costs add up to just a fraction of what you would have to pay in lump sum to get that car operating again in the unlikely event of a breakdown.

This concept also holds true in the Construction field as well. With proper planning, time and money is saved. Profits can grow. Without proper planning, time and money is wasted. Removing, reshaping, and redoing become additional expenses and cuts profits. A correct understanding of food and nutrition provides a blueprint, much like how an architect draws out the plan for a building. When we follow the guidelines of correct foods and good nutrition, we save time and money, and add value to our life. Good health and proper construction techniques have a lot in common. Proper planning, selection and use of the best materials, and enjoying the wealth of the functioning product is the overall aim and objective of every body and project.

These examples could teach us a lot about the human body and how it functions. When we feed our bodies proper nutrients, we experience a human body working at its best. Everything works and feels better. Our cells are well fed and flowing with energy. We feel more alive and live more active lives. Exercise comes naturally. That down and out feeling would be a thing of the past simply because the brain and the body now has more energy and operates in more favorable conditions.

It all starts with thinking positive and valuable thoughts about ourselves. We can literally will ourselves into good health and longevity when we choose to. Once there is emphasis on *who* and *why* we are, then the tendency to think more consciously happens naturally. The things within and around us, and how they affect us, naturally grow in importance. The mind creates the environment where more positive thoughts can flow through, activating these parts of our brain which were previously sleeping or clouded. Now we can think more correctly. Like I told you earlier, there is no real mystery to this. It is instead natural science.

Now that we have cleared away some of the dust that was rusting and clouding our better judgment, we start paying more interest and attention to ourselves. We now begin to understand that everything is really connected and indeed one does affect the other. We start recognizing the brighter side of life instead of the one that keeps us frustrated and in fear. We start reading the ingredients on packaged products, and we start asking questions at the grocery store and at the farmer's market.

The need to know now becomes more important to us and our power of observation grows. Our mental faculties begin to blossom and bloom. These natural reactions point to a path where we now seek to protect and preserve (as much as possible) this precious opportunity that we have been granted called Life. Not only of our own but that of our loved ones and those around us also. Within this reality our magnetic field glows and good energy flows into our minds, bodies, and souls. If there is any doubt in your mind, all you need to do is to try it. Experience natural food therapy and live happy.

In no way am I suggesting any form of extremism here. I am talking about a natural and gradual process occurring within and around us. The process has always been ongoing. However it is now your time to get in tune with it and open up doors to greater consciousness. The journey of Life does take a turn for the better at this point. Good food taste great and give life. Instead of being blind and unaware of that which affects us, we now begin to understand how products are put together. We also begin to study their positive or negative effects. We naturally develop a certain discipline within ourselves which is truly one with our natural being. Life is a joy and we should live it thankfully. What fun is there in spending most of our productive life suffering from aches and pains? These discomforts could be simply avoided by increasing our own knowledge in the field of natural health consciousness.

Some of us spend the majority of our life savings fighting cruel diseases which could have been avoided. *Food Politricks* is here to help us be more aware of the effects of what we eat and call food. It may seem a bit strange to think that it is not in the best interests of the majority of "Health Care Practitioners" to educate the public about how to maintain better healthcare practices. It is more profitable to these health experts to prescribe aesthetic drugs to the public than to teach us how to keep ourselves in proper health and living conditions. The fact of the matter is, the medical industry focuses on the Treatment of diseases, not on the Prevention of diseases.

Doctors and other medical practitioners are trained to treat sickness and diseases. They are not in the business of Education for Prevention of disease. They are in the business of DRUG Add-ministration! And the funny thing about these prescription drugs are their side effects. They claim to fix one issue while causing other areas of the body to malfunction. Then more drugs are prescribed for these new diseases and this detrimental cycle continues until the end. Not of the disease mind you, but of the person trying to stay alive.

After so many weeks or months, the prescription has to be renewed and often the dosage increased. There is always a steady flow of revenue through these medical doctors on to the pharmaceutical companies and their affiliates. Be informed here and now that sick persons are often used as "guinea pigs" while these biochemists have their sales representatives test out new drugs. They want to find out which one works best and what are the side effects. Instead of being used as a tool to full the cash registers of these multi billion dollar corporations, why not claim responsible for your own health, wellness, and prosperity?

It is now up to us as individuals and families to begin to reeducate ourselves. It is now time to equip ourselves with the correct tools necessary for gaining more knowledge in identifying and maintaining better health habits. If we allow the cycle to continue where other people are responsible for our own health care, we will always remain victims to a health care system that is not designed as I said earlier to educate us. Therefore, health education should be a serious topic during family discussions, and a subject in all forms of mandatory educational institutions of learning – from kindergarten to university; and even in every church!

Give us the opportunity to grow up with a sense of knowing how valuable good health is to any and every aspect of our Life. It does not matter what your hopes and dreams are, or what denomination you may align yourself to. Without good health no one will ever be able to achieve goals or success for any sustained period of time. In reality, our chances of fulfilling our goals and achieving our dreams depend on how healthy we are to perform what ever we need to in order to accomplish our missions.

This is what this book is really about. It is an opportunity for those of us who have made this simple yet powerful transformation within ourselves to gain strength. It is also for those of us who are thinking about making certain changes and need help as to which way to go. Believe me when I say that you are not alone. We are all looking to expand our experience. We are interested in knowing more as to the variety of menu options open to us.

It is often thought that when one decides to eat from a healthier menu, starvation and death is sure to follow. Most of your peers may tell you that if you choose not to eat animal flesh and/or dairy products for instance, you basically have nothing left to eat. This is a total misconception and a basic product of our upbringing. Most of us were fed this animal parts and dairy diet as a child. The idea of eating without the consumption of animal flesh and dairy for example, has never been truly thought of, far less to be explored and introduced into our families and societies. Well it actually has, but that subject is for a next chapter or a next book altogether.

Is it a matter of teachings and conditioning? It is unlikely that you will learn about anything that you are not taught or been exposed to. There is the need for true education. We need to be exposed to and taught different and alternative ideas than what is being presently advertized. In that way we would be in a better position to make decisions, since the pool of knowledge and choice would be much greater. I know for a fact that no parent would willingly prepare a meal for their child, knowing definitely that this meal could potentially hurt their child. Parents go through extreme measures to take care of and protect their children. We would not personally serve destructive meals with 'love' would we? This idea is totally crazy! Therefore, it is in the line of education that barriers to knowledge are always broken.

We would learn that there is no shortage of natural fruits, grains, nuts, beans, herbs, and vegetables on this planet. We would learn that feeding cows for human consumption requires more natural resources than humans feeding on nature for ourselves. We would also learn that there are numerous options, recipes, and products that exist naturally, have been created, and can be created from this wealth of natural resources that we have. That is the focus of the second part of this book. These recipes are very simple and do not include rare ingredients that are hard to find.

It seems to me that some one has taken it upon themselves to spread the propaganda that natural living, cooking, eating, etc. is difficult and stressful. It should not be this way and I am happy to say that in reality, it is not that way. Most natural things around us are important and very valuable to our life and health. Have you ever considered the fact that we receive our much needed oxygen from the growing trees? And that these trees produce this life giving oxygen from the carbon dioxide that we exhale to them? Have you ever taken a moment to truly consider this amazing relationship?

Modernization has taken us away from our ancient menu which was such an important part of our culture. Nature keeps us strong, healthy, and free from diseases! Mental Colonization has forced most of us into a lifestyle of fast food, artificial flavors and colorings, chemical preservatives and additives. As a result, the quality of our health has been rapidly decreasing at a very alarming rate. Our great grand parents never knew what a sprite or a chubby was. They never ate at fast food restaurants like KFC, McDonalds, or Burger King.

They also never suffered from cancer, diabetes, strokes, and obesity, etc. at the rate that plague nations today.

We came from a culture founded on herbs, grains, nuts, vegetables, fruits, provisions, and spring clean water. We paid such close attention to nature to the point where we could tell when it was going to rain by simply looking at the sky, or feeling the change in temperature of the wind. We knew how to utilize our environment for the benefit of the community. We were respected simply because of the significant contributions that we made towards the general progress and livelihood of our people. We were also a more active people with our work consisting mostly of agriculture, trades, skilled labor, etc. There were not so many offices where people were encouraged to sit down to work. The "couch potato syndrome" would be quite a strange occurrence to our great grand parents. Such a lifestyle would be unimaginable.

In the more industrialized nations there are hardly any backyard gardens. There are a few states here and there known for farming and agriculture, but that's it. So many have never seen how a pumpkin or a potato grows. In the Caribbean Islands and other tropical areas like Africa, and South and Central America however, there are a huge variety of herbs, beans, nuts, fruits, vegetables, and root crops etc. This range of assorted supply contains together, every nutrient known to feed cells and organs. This formula maintains a better nutrient balance and encourages true health.

Our ancestors lived on this simple menu. The results have given us real evidence as in the life of our now famous Ma Pampo, who lived well past one hundred and twenty five (125) years on the Nature Island of Waiti Kubuli (Dominica). Many Centenarians have lived and are still living on my island.

As a matter of fact, this island called Dominica has the most Centenarians per capita than any where else in the world. I wonder why? Keep in mind that the colonizers refer to this part of the earth as third world and under-developed. Yet the developed world has yet to produce many - especially on a consistent basis - living past the age of even 90 years old. Shouldn't the so called "first world" nations be way more advanced in terms of healthcare and longevity than a bunch of poor third world islands?

Love your life and learn how to take better care of yourself. Life was created for us to live long and happy lives. Choose life. Do not be tricked into buying and eating yourself away. Reclaim possession of your life, health, and strength. Please do. We all have a choice to make.

The Myth vs. Reality

There is this old time saying that you are what you eat! Many people might argue and say no way. Ok. So you may not actually be what you eat literally, but what you eat definitely influences how you live and your health in general. To be in good health means to be happy; free from stress, aches, pains, dis-ease, and dis-comforts. What joy is life if you are constantly in agony and pain? No one likes feeling sick. Yet, too often we find ourselves or someone we know admitted to the hospitals, health centers, and doctor's offices; only to find them packed with lines longer than when we go to the bank.

We need to truly investigate the root of these diseases and do our best to prevent them from taking further control of us and our nations. My investigation thus far has led me to the conclusion that we should pay more attention to the foods that we eat. We should spend a little more time reading these labels, and actually look up the meaning of these chemical ingredients dumped in foods as additives, artificial flavorings, and preservatives. These toxins are being pumped into the majority of processed foods which the nations of the world consume on a daily basis.

In passing, could it be that third world countries are labeled as such because of Economic and Mental poverty? If this is so, we can get rid off mental and economic poverty when there is an Awakening as to the real concepts securing good health. We can then build our own wealth and create more opportunities to stamp out all forms of poverty. How can this become reality? Minds and eyes need to open up to view the reality of Food Security. Let me remind you that Food is the Staff of Life; the lifeline of any nation. It is time to wake up from the sleep and slumber! *"Arise ye mighty peo-*

ple. Accomplish what you will". These thundering words from the visionary prophet Marcus Garvey ring louder today than ever before. Let us believe and create our own miracles.

At this point in time I would like to make this announcement; "we need to take this slogan seriously – say no to DRUGS!" The dictionary actually defines drugs as any substance that acts on the nervous system. It also seemed odd to me that in America and throughout the developed world, Food and Drugs are controlled and regulated by the same agency. This agency responsible for food authenticity, its quality and content, is the Food and Drug Administration or the FDA. This may sound strange, but it is very true. Processed foods have to pass through this agency. They are ones responsible for determining the shelf life of consumer food and drug products. They are the ones who give the expiration date found on most of the stock sold in the supermarkets and stores. This date is calculated based on the strength of the chemical substance acting as the preservative. Think about it for a minute.

If you were to actually research the chemical makeup of some of these ingredients, you would be amazed. There are words that literarily cannot be pronounced. There are those sometimes not even found in dictionary. Some are not even found on the internet for that matter. You would need a medical encyclopedia to get the meaning of some of these. It is time to start seriously saying NO to these Drugs. These additives are inorganic and unnatural. These are the substances mostly responsible for eventual cell and organ malfunction, and the weakening of the overall immune and nervous systems. This catastrophe leaves the organs open to the germs that cause influenza (the flu), sickness, chronic diseases, and eventually death.

Another serious issue to look at is the topic of the ever popular 'white meat' known as chicken. Growing up we came to know the fowls in the yards and neighborhoods. The fact is that it seemed like years before they were ready for the pot. These fowls ate corn, coconut, a local plant we call zeb gwa (fat grass), and things of that sort. They were free to move about, and knew exactly what tree to climb to go to bed at evening time. These were the earliest alarm clocks.

Nowadays you have a fast food chicken being chemically manufactured at a disturbing rate to keep up with the demands of a chicken addicted world. These ready-made chickens are force-fed through needles in their veins. Have you noticed the little hole at the top of the drumstick? Huge amounts of steroids, estrogen, and other growth hormones make them ready for consumption in approximately six (6) weeks or less from the egg! How interesting is that?

These organisms are reared specifically for the market and are victims of severe stress. They become chemically imbalanced as a result of their torture through this horrible mass production process. When someone feasts on these mechanical chickens, these dangerous steroids and growth enhancing hormones are also ingested. The more often someone eats these lab created organisms, the sooner it is that their body will begin to show evidence of malfunction in many different ways. Our great grand parents are really shaking their heads by now on this one.

Have you ever noticed how young children develop so

quickly, especially in these "first world" countries? Pre teen-age girls have started their menstrual cycles and are walking around with breasts. This would be considered abnormal back in the day for their age. More strangely, even boys are growing "breasts" these days. Another significant observation is the current rise in cases of fibroids. This is a relatively new phenomenon that medical practitioners are claiming they don't know what is causing the growth of these dangerous organisms that occupy the most sensitive areas of a woman's womb.

Presently in Dominica and in the entire Caribbean for that matter, fibroids are almost an epidemic! Thousands of young women and even older ladies are complaining of severe discomfort in the womb area, hemorrhaging, irregular menstrual cycles, and even barrenness. Many of these women have already undergone surgery, which they are told have to be repeated after some years. Some have even had their entire wombs removed! While medical doctors claim they are uncertain as to what is really causing fibroids, they are making millions of dollars performing operations. They scrape the lining of the womb or cut off the bigger fibroid leaving the smaller ones behind to continue growing.

Do your own research. The fibroid is a living bacterial organism which occupies itself within the tissues in and around the ovaries and uterus. They compete for space and nutrients. It is about time Medical researchers do some serious investigations into the evident relationship between these new diseases and this trend of mass-produced chicken, meat and dairy products, and overall fast food consumption. Is it really a mystery? Is it a willful attack against the nations of the world? The burning question flares on, gaining momentum around every corner.

Some years ago we were introduced to a strange outbreak termed as Mad Cow disease. You only have to visit a cattle farm for yourself or check up on the behind the scenes to understand why these cows would grow insane. Their rearing conditions are terrible! In addition to this, we are aware that cows are and have always been eaters of grass from the beginning of cow time. It is rather mind boggling to learn that dead cows and other animals were being ground into meal and fed to these cattle. No wonder these cows lost their brains! This change from natural diet tampered with the very engineering of the cow's infrastructure. They literally went off their hinges.

Now can you imagine what happens to humans who continue to ingest the meat of such animals? All the torture and stress that goes into the slaughtering of these animals could never result in a product that would be healthy for human consumption. All this being said, the FDA grades and places an approved label on such produce, making them now safe and permissible to be distributed near, far, and wide. The worst and lowest grades make their way to Africa, the Caribbean, South and Central America, and other so called third world countries. Is this by coincidence? I don't think so. Do you?

Pork isn't being treated any better. The same principal of torture applies. Eating and consuming these stress infested produce will continue to lead to all forms of hormonal imbalances, organ dysfunction, tumors, cancers, and numerous other health complications too much to mention here. Our leaders really need to take a deeper look into this meat and poultry industry and strive for better ways and means to supply the nation with more health conscious options.

The management of the nation's affairs should also become more attentive to another very important fact. The use of poisons such as gramaxone, mocap, round up etc; and chemical fertilizers in agriculture are extremely hazardous to human health. These dangerous chemicals kill out most of the life in the soil, including the natural minerals and other trace elements, by seriously infecting the soil with poisonous chemicals. Most farmers actually replant seedlings and other plants in these contaminated soils, and then sell this as food to the public for consumption. Some of these produce nowadays are being grown from a seed or seedlings that have already been implanted with in-grown pesticides. These are extremely harmful to the human nervous and immune systems.

What then happens to the local vegetables and ground provisions which should be chosen above processed and imported foods? To put it simply, "contaminated soils produce contaminated produce/food. These poisons eventually find their way into the streams and rivers, infecting the water supply, causing further damage to us. Are you one of those still wondering where all the mountain chicken, crayfish, vieyo (a snail looking shelled animal stuck on to the river stones), and river crabs disappeared to? A large number of women are discovering that they are suffering from fibroids, and that they may even be barren. Men are now suffering from baldness, prostate cancer, and impotence at very early ages. Whoever said you are what you eat, really knew what they were talking about.

The way forward: "Back to the Future"

It may sound strange to you, but our great grand parents knew what they were dealing with, more than we seem to know now even with all our modern technology. If you were to compare, they lived stronger lives despite the daily slavery required of them. They were put through much physical labor, with sometimes no real leisure time, and yet they lived longer stronger lives than modern day people who basically work less and have more free time. Is there a lesson here? Did it have something to do with the food that they ate?

My great great grand mothers and fathers were taken from Africa with the knowledge of our ancestors. It would seem that their "hard work" kept them strong, active and healthy. Or was it the herbs and the food that they were eating? Today we work less, have more leisure time, eat more, do fewer exercises, and are more diseased than they ever were. They were robbed of their rights to live as free people, but they had the knowledge of our culture. Our path has been always cut along the course of Nature!

We are connected to the earth – Mother Nature, who is the Mother of us all. She provides great tidings, all nutrients, vitamins and minerals for our life. She contains in her bosom all ingredients for all living beings on this planet. Mother Nature has never stopped producing varieties of fresh fruits, grains, nuts, herbs, provisions, vegetables, etc. sufficient to feed all her children and keep us in great health. This ancient culture of feeding from Nature's sources has been in existence ever since the very beginning of time.

Like a mother is responsible for feeding her young, similarly, so is the earth responsible for feeding her us. It has been proven and we now know for a fact that a mother's breast milk is best for her babies. It contains all natural nutrients sufficient to feed and grow the young child. Similarly, Mother Nature contains within her offerings every nutrient known to sustain balance, and maintain the proper function of every organ in the human structure. Sickness and diseases occur when organs and other controlling systems lack sufficient nutrition to function with ease. Without the life giving substances found in real and correct foods, these organs go out of their natural balance. This is when germs, toxins, and disease take over.

Artificial substances may seem similar to the natural substances, but they are *definitely not the same.* Great marketing campaigns attract us into believing that the chemical components are just as good as the natural occurring elements. They preach that we miss nothing *really* when we substitute. Most of these chemical compounds and additives are inorganic substances that offer no nutritional benefit to the cells of the human body. On the contrary, they actually do the opposite. Incorrect foods take energy from the cells, breaking them down and paving the way for germs, bacteria, viruses, and fungus to grow and take control. Many who fell for these marketing strategies have already paid with their life. Some are paying the price presently with pain and sickness. This trend will continue as long as ignorance of the truth continues to exist.

We need to equalize the playing field. The time has come for research and reeducation. Pharmaceutical companies pour millions of dollars into research and development for the drugs and other chemical substances they produce. They produce a market ready product well labeled with ingredients and nutritional information down to percentage points. They create commercials and contract the best persons possible to market their products. Massive campaigns are run through the various media houses, and these companies make certain that their product and message reach the minds of as many people as possible. These corporations follow a comprehensive plan and they execute this plan down to the very last cent.

Natural health care companies and groups need to grow to the point where we can also invest and implement the same strategies in Natural Health Care products and services. The major difference would be that our plans and products would be designed to add joy and health to life. We would be able to experiment with dandelion and Aloe Vera leaves for instance, and analyze all their major components and active ingredients. We would know the content of the life giving properties contained in an avocado, spinach, and sweet potato. We would be able to determine the amount of a particular substance necessary to alleviate (targeted) cell stress, reverse the diseased state, and maintain perfect health from that time forward. This is Natural science in full effect.

We would be able to conduct experiments documenting and proving the Truth living inside so many of these life saving plants. No longer would Herbology (the study of living herbs) be looked at as a myth or an unnecessary science. We would begin to realize that this is actually the oldest science and reality that there is. Instead of continuing as the mystery it has been reduced to, the study behind the magic of Herbal Medicine would become a subject at home, at school, at church, and at play.

Those of us who till the soil would also become more

knowledgeable as to the great importance of true agriculture and take pride in it. No longer would the soil be poisoned before planting. We would learn to look at the earth as sacred ground and look at ourselves as caretakers of this beautiful paradise. We would contribute positively to our own life and the lives of as many as we feed. The vibration of wisdom, love and unity would grow. We would become more connected to each other. To recognize similarities amongst ourselves would be easier to achieve than to stay trapped fighting differences. We would recognize that we are truly one earth family and that it has never been all about me, myself, and I.

We are living in a time where all knowledge is basically at our finger tips. Anything we want to know about anyone or anything is available within seconds with the correct tools and networks. Yet we know so little about these life generating resources known as living plants and their life giving properties. The reality is that our entire existence depends on these green trees. It would be now scientifically proven and the documented evidence left for generations to come, that there is contained within these natural food sources, life saving and sustaining nutrients. We would also know at what dosage to apply these miracles of knowledge. There would no longer be uncertainty as to the authenticity of herbs and natural food. The nations of the world would be able to live much healthier and fulfilled lives. Families and friends would once again work together for the common prosperity of all.

In order to live in glory, happiness, and honor, we first have to recognize that we are indeed each others keepers. Once we ascend to that point, we simply follow nature's benevolent laws and live always and forever. Remember to be thankful for everything. In everything give thanks.

The Science of Food

Most of us are currently uncomfortable with how we feel, how we look, our energy levels, our self esteem, etc. The basic truth is that in most cases, artificial food will do that to you. The science of food states that natural sources of food contain trace elements and other vital minerals that these chemical foods could never contain. Also natural substances in proper proportions do not produce side effects. We cannot say the same for chemical foods. While they appear harmless, filling the stomach and satisfying hunger, they may be damaging our cells and vital organs.

In his important little book titled "Dr. Frank's No Aging Diet", Dr. Benjamin S. Frank had this to say. *Good health is the natural state of the human body. I believe in maintaining this state - and in restoring it if it is lost - in ways that are natural to the body: not with powerful drugs but with natural nutrients. I have found that these nutrients work better and are far safer than medicines which are so powerful (the word should really be dangerous) that the public must be protected from them by laws that require prescriptions... Of course, everyone agrees that good nutrition is essential to good health. However, my research shows that it can be far more effective than was ever suspected, not only in maintaining good health but in restoring it when disease sets in... What's more, these diseases spring from the same root cause. Treat the root cause of one and you are treating the root cause of the others."*

Scientist, chemists, and other medical experts are well aware that the real teacher is Mother Nature. Most experiments are based on arriving as close to the natural substance as possible. The following result is only an imitation. We need to be made aware of these facts also. There is great danger in moving away from nature to adopt a more artificial culture. The results can be very deadly as we are seeing today. Just take a look at the lines at the hospitals and health centers around your area. The lines are longer than those at the bank! Many people work their entire life only to end up spending their life savings seeking medical attention.   Most go to the grave in debt. Talk about irony.

We were gifted by the Almighty with healthy bodies and functioning minds. However, we are born into a world where we are encouraged to trade in our healthy bodies for material possessions. Whatever we cannot afford to purchase outright, we are encouraged to loan and credit. Why don't we spend some of this money eating the best foods available? At the end of the journey we leave all these material possessions behind while we lay suffering. Our health decreases down the road to death and destruction, and no amount of money in this world can bring us back to life.

It's almost like the story of the dog that lost its bone, only on a much greater scale. In this situation the dog actually loses its life! I think we all want to live long, joyful, fruitful lives, as far away from pain and diseases as possible. Sadly however, most of us don't know where to begin to understand who we really are, why we really are, and how exactly do we approach fulfilling our true purpose and healthy destiny.

I think that there is need for a road map. Some form of guideline other than the _Basic Instruction Before Leaving Earth_, is necessary. Or better yet, we need an example of someone or groups of people who have actually got to the level of life we hope so much to achieve. We also need to study our own ancestors and our culture! At one point in time, though Africans were considered slaves by the oppressors, we were healthy enough to ask these "masters" why were they sick? We did not really understand what was going on. To our great grand parents, sickness was a very unfamiliar concept. When we got sick we knew the natural remedy. As twisted as history can sometimes be, it still says that some oppressors would be healed simply by placing their bare feet on the back of a "slave". The very DNA and structure of our bodies at that time, though far removed from our natural environment, was still strong and well nourished enough to perform such miracles. Could you imagine what miracles we could perform today? Who knows? Is it too late to find out? Time will tell.

Like I said before, we only need to truly investigate our own culture, and we will discover that even to this day we have on the Nature Island of Dominica a great number of centenarians who are quite mobile. These are perfect examples that life is for the living. They are survivors from that great culture who understood much more than we seem to know now about the Laws of Nature and how well they operate within and around our human system. It is quite evident that most of us today have moved away from our ancient menu culture of roast provision and cashew nuts, fruits, greens, and herbal teas. Most of us are now caught up in a money spending web created by pharmaceutical companies and processed food manufacturers.

These corporations use their grand marketing campaigns to continually influence and captivate the minds of the public into believing that their artificial way of chemicals and drugs is the best way to go. Once again I would like to repeat that those who fall for these advertisements also fall victim to bad health and malfunction. Those of us who live the happiest and longest are sometimes those who cannot afford to purchase those pretty packages of junk food.

The science of food comes down to this. To fully comprehend the relationship between man, health, and the food we eat, we need to feed as closely as possible from that menu which nature prescribes. We have had years of feasting on artificial and processed foods. We have seen the damage over the years and there are too many statistics and death announcements to prove it. Many people have gone across to the other side of life earlier that later simply because they were ignorant of the nutritional facts that truly govern their life. Health and nutrition should be taught in every school and church. Every institution of learning should be teaching students how to live a healthier life. What does life truly depends on? The hustle and bustle of employment, bills, and survival has taken it toll on the best of us. The quality of food that we eat becomes of such important that this message cannot be overemphasized. We are what we eat!

We have no more time it seems to seek the truly important treasures of life. Instead most of us work to pay bills and purchase the latest products on the consumer market. Major companies generate billions of dollars while so many people are growing sick and dying. The populations of the world have been reduced to mere consumers. All is fair in the game of profit they say. But what do you say?

The science of food reminds us of who we are and where we truly came from. This concept encourages us to know ourselves, to be wise, and to live in accordance with the laws of nature. Eat healthy and live happy. It is time we all came back home to the one who has always loved us. Oh Mother Nature, how bountiful are your presents?

From Agriculture to Disaster

Decide for yourself. It is becoming more and more apparent that the promoters of the artificial world are raging a serious war against nature and natural healers. Or are they really? The facts are as follows.

Look at the way that food is being planted for human consumption. It has become common practice for farmers to spray the ground with gramaxone and other deadly poisons in preparation for planting instead of weeding the old fashion way. The area is then cleared, and after a short time, seeds, seedlings, and other plants are planted in these toxic soils. Then the farmers complain that their crops are not doing so well. So they go to the store or to the government for chemical fertilizers to boost the depleted condition of the soil.

These days while some crops like bananas and plantains are growing, farmers get rid of the weeds growing around them by using pesticides and other dangerous chemicals. While these produce grows, they also feed on their polluted environment. This happens even if this process is not visible to the naked eye. However, when you look at the number of farmers who have suffered and died from respiratory problems, bladder and kidney malfunction, and prostate cancer in the past twenty to thirty years, the statistics are unbelievable! It is quite interesting to me. Professionals in the agricultural field should see this obvious connection between these toxins called pesticides and chemicals called fertilizers; and the effect that they have on human health conditions. Organic agriculture is the answer to so many of our current health problems!

Most foods sold in the supermarket today are genetically modified and engineered. These foods are being created in a laboratory. This is definitely not the best for a human system that is created totally natural. The raw materials for these products are grown under controlled, laboratory environments. The very seed has been modified from start to be able to resist certain diseases. Pesticides have already been injected into these seed's embryos. These seedlings appear to grow into healthy products well suited for the food processing factories and on to the supermarkets. It would seem that these large corporations appear to be more interested in the way the produce looks, the short time needed for maturity, and their market price; than in the human benefit of these food substances.

For the profit of these chemical companies, supermarkets chains, and other involved in the generating end of the cycle, these toxins get processed into foods and flood the markets of even the lesser developed countries. The best grades are considered for these industrial and technological countries, while the worst of the categories go to the places classified as third world. Small farmers are becoming dependent on chemicals; from seeds, to pesticides, and then to fertilizers. They spend more time and money trying to return some of the natural elements of the soils that were destroyed during the poisonous preparation process. This I term as reverse or poverty economics - a dangerous situation plaguing the African Continent, the Caribbean Islands, and the rest of the poorer nations. The time has come to do something about it.

Compare the two. Organic farming has been the foundation of agriculture from ever since creation began. Our ancestors knew nothing about miracle grow or round up. Long before these major corporations and their products, our great parents knew when to plant, what to plant, where, why, and how. They also had natural ways and means to maintain the soil mineral content by using crop rotation techniques and natural fertilizers like compost, ashes, etc. They never used gramaxone. They also did not suffer from some of the majority of diseases that so many suffer from today. Most were free from respiratory problems, heart complications, cancers, and the host of other CNDCs killing out the human family as we speak. They lived healthier stronger lives.

This outbreak of Chronic Non-Communicable Diseases (or CNCD's as they are commonly termed), have been closely and directly linked to diet according to a recent study by the World Health Organization (WHO). They also confirmed that *"...even if there was consensus that the unhealthy diet of refined processed foods, meat consumption, and dairy products has been identified as the major cause of these illnesses, the trend towards a healthier diet will not be implemented because the owners of these large corporate entities stand to lose too much.* I am beginning to understand the real truth behind the quote, *"...for the love of money, is the root of all evil!"* As long as people keep on purchasing these products, these companies will continue to supply this demand with their chemicals. The sales of these chemical products and processed foods bring in billions of dollars a year in revenue to these companies and their share holders. The sick and dying spend billions trying to regain their health. Who are the ones really benefiting from this cycle?

According to the WHO, *CNCD's will cost the planet about two hundred and thirty eight (238) Billion dollars in the next few years. This pandemic is directly linked to poor nutrition and this SAD (Standard American Diet) that the peoples of the world are currently indulging themselves in.* What we are seeing here is the total opposite of the way things used to be for our Great Grand parents. They knew not of these devils so nicely packaged in plastics, cans, jars, bottles, and boxes. Mother Earth has provided and sustained our culture and livity (way of life) for millennia! Nature has fed us properly from ever since the beginning of time. We should be so very thankful.

Most parents these days have been tricked into a deadly scheme through million dollar advertising campaigns as previously mentioned. Powerful media houses have been properly paid to ensure that these ads blast on the airwaves – promoting their latest products. A family outing at KFC or McDonald's is the order of the day. Junk food neatly packaged (read the ingredients) are sold in these huge grocery (grow sorry) stores, and this is what stock the kitchen cupboards of the majority of homes. I am not saying that we should not purchase anything from the stores. What I am suggesting is that we make healthier choices when we go out food shopping.

Snack time now includes something like Coca Cola, Busta, Chubby, and other soft drinks; and Doritos or Lay's potato chips for example. Gone are the days of an orange or a banana. There is no wonder why the rate of obesity is past alarming. The bell has been ringing for some years now. No one who is "somebody" seems to be paying any attention and the situation is now way past out-of-control! We *need* to do something about it before it really gets too late.

Agriculture is the greatest culture ever. It not only feeds and sustains our life, but it is also creates and supports a *culture* where we can all *agree*. Even small children have important roles to play in the process. Many hands make light the work has been a true and proven fact. All who are involved in the process receives a feeling of accomplishment when the produce reaches maturity. To eat something that you have planted, nurtured, and watch grow into readiness is an extremely unique experience. You should try it. Everyone involved feels happy and an important part of the whole life giving process.

However, when we move away from the close relationship with mother earth and particularly agriculture, we also become further removed from the natural state of our own mind and health. Other ideas and means of survival have to be practiced which is usually not as wholesome and life generating as being involved in direct agriculture. A serious solution to the numerous life threatening issues facing most of the earth's youth today can be solved with a general shift towards true agriculture.

Many young people do not understand that it takes time for things to grow and mature. Too many walk around with the concept that everything in life is instant like coffee and Google. Agriculture would help them to understand that patience in indeed one of the highest virtues. Put your mind towards a particular goal and stick to it. In time, with determination, patience, and wise choices, you will achieve your goals. Try it for yourself. Agriculture is natural health therapy.

.

The Conspiracy

In between time, thousands of us are losing our lives daily through diseases that could have simply been avoided through proper nutrition and sufficient exercise. Loved ones experience tremendous loss emotionally and financially everyday, because of a true knowledge of which we are being systematically deprived. It is more profitable for these pharmaceutical corporations to treat diseases rather than to prevent them. Treatment of diseases generate trillions of dollars for a few while bringing debt, suffering, and death to multitudes. Are these notorious few the ones responsible for leading the other ninety percent (98%) down that road of total destruction? If so be the case, you can see why the words "for the love of money is the root of all evil" ring so true. It seems that monetary profit for a few is more important than the lives of billions of people.

There is a serious quote in Dr. Beiler's book *Food Is Your Best Medicine* stating, *"The aim of medicine is to prevent disease and prolong life; the ideal of medicine is to eliminate the need for a physician" (words of Dr. William J. Mayo, M.D.)* I take it that the persons who own and operate these big drug corporations were absent from school on that day. Instead, millions of dollars are being spent on Research and Development for treatment of diseases that could simply be avoided by living and eating naturally. The same funding could be put into education and promotion of Natural Healthcare programs! To understand how the natural human body truly functions in relation with nature – Mother to us all – would benefit everyone living on this planet. All cells grow alive and well whenever there is sufficient nutrients and oxygen. Health goes hand in hand with cleanliness. Cleanliness is Godliness! Health and

GOD walk hand in hand. Get the message.

Once again I say, there is no real mystery to this. The answer is right in front of our faces. All we need to do is to take a good look, within and around ourselves. Individuals and families in general would learn to be more in tune with each other and the surroundings. Instead of being stuck to a couch or fixed to a television screen consuming junk food, we could be out breathing in fresh air, exercising, and exploring the earth.

When was the last time you took a nature walk adventure? You would discover new things and be asking yourself new questions. These questions bring home some very interesting new answers. Knowledge increases naturally, rewarding and giving strength to all who participate. Health and longevity does not only depend on what we eat. It also involves our consciousness and awareness. To know that the ability to live a full life or suffer with pain and death is determined by the food choices we make everyday is truly an amazing thought. Think about this concept. The right choice is crystal clear but most of us are being convinced daily to ruin our health. We do this at our own free will (under heavy influence), three and four times a day and sometimes even more.

It seems strange that the same agency and corporation responsible for food quality, control, and security is also the same agency responsible for the approval of pharmaceutical drugs and other chemicals found in food. Is the FDA (the Food and Drug Addministration) the medium whereby these destructive and deadly chemicals or DRUGS get into our food supply? It is a question worth asking since we are seeing this current trend of genetically modified food (GM Foods) and artificial flavorings responsible for causing death to so many.

Pills and poisons are currently replacing natural food as we know it! Would there ever be an objective to kill out billions of people through simple, unnecessary, "natural causes" of death? In other words, is there a strategy aimed at mass population reduction? Is the Food and Drug Administration the vehicle driving this multi level trillion dollar pharmaceutical/drug industry? Why would an agency be approving dangerous chemicals destined for human consumption? This idea is very hard to digest. Yet reality speaks so clear.

Read the Labels! I cannot say that enough. When you do you will be surprised as I was as to the extent that these corporations go to ensure that you get sick. Remember this; a healthy person is of no benefit to either the medical professionals or to the pharmaceutical companies. The only people important to these professionals are those of us whose health is decreasing. We are the ones who become important targets to these drug lords and they jump on us as opportunities. They use our misfortune as their opportunity to introduce us to their variety of medications and services that could solve our problems.

Fear walks alongside diseases. Now these campaigns become interesting. The next thing you know, some of us purchase these products or agree to the service which is usually a surgical operation. The patient now becomes a victim to the many follow up programs and additional experimental drugs which these companies have to offer for sale. Then comes in the ever present companion of these drugs; their side effects. A patient is reduced to a high paying customer. The greater the ailment, the more profitable we become to these companies. More patients translate into higher profits for these corporations and to them that's good business.

Thus, it is part of the packaging and the scheme to make certain that as many of us as possible gets sick. That is where the very important FDA comes in. Through skilled lobbyists working on behalf of their employers, large donations are made to this agency to keep things rolling the way of the corporations. Like I mentioned before, even the WHO agreed that even if there was consensus; things would not change. The reality of *Food Politricks* comes down to a game of business and billion dollar profits.

You may have never thought of things in this way, but the super markets and grocery stores become the store houses and money generating outlets for these chemicals packaged so nicely in processed foods. People unconsciously go to the stores and purchase chemically imbalanced foods that will eventually make them sick. Parents feed these foods to their children and after some time they too become sick and have to visit the doctor as well. This viscous cycle has been going on for years, generating billions of dollars annually in revenue for these huge corporations. These companies share large dividends while millions of people suffer and die every year from diseases and complications. I guess its all in the game huh? Good GOD Almighty!

The time is at hand. Since in the 1970s the call was made to grow what you eat and eat what you grow. While we are on this subject, please take some time to educate yourself on the ingredients that you eat. Chemicals substances are now being termed as food. For example, do you really know what mono sodium glutamate (MSG) is? What effects does it have on the human brain and health in general? The truth of the matter is this; what you don't know can literally kill you and at an expensive price as well. The reality and fact of the situation is this; as long as we continue to buy and eat these chemicals, we will continue to die from the effects these chemicals working against our health and wellness.

Rewiring Our Circuits

The ingredients are right there on the package and most people never even take the time out to read what it is that they are about to eat. Food feeds the cells responsible for our own health and life. Have you ever found out what Red #40 is? Or Blue #6? Did you find out what are the components of MSG (mono sodium glutamate)? What keeps the red bloody meat looking so fresh though this animal has been slaughtered for months and even years? Some will say they don't have time for that. Some reach as far as saying that "they are living and they must die, so they don't really care that much..." Too late, too late is usually their cry when that time comes. The mere fact that you are reading these words mean that even *now*, you can start making some necessary positive changes in your food choices and life in general. Your friends might look at you strangely at first until they themselves start seeing the difference in you and begin to understand the benefits of making healthier choices. So my friend you can be a spark and an example. Go for it!

Just the other day I heard a story of two coworkers. There was one who was more health conscious, bringing her home cooked meals to work for lunch. The other was very satisfied with buying regular lunch meals filled with starch, meat, high salt, and fats. As a matter of fact, the coworker who buys lunch often made fun of her coworker for trying to be too health conscious. Well what do you know? One day the buying coworker came to work and collapse. Who was there to her rescue? If you said the health conscious coworker, you are very correct. This may not always be the case, but it is a perfect example of the current state of affairs where health is concerned.

Those who don't care and feel that what we eat is of little importance to our overall well-being will be the ones suffering. Those of us who try to help our bodies help itself will definitely reap the benefits of a richer and more fulfilled life. So many children today never get to spend good quality time with their grandparents, all because grandma and grandpa are not in good health. Even some parents have difficulty having fun with their children because fatigue and obesity has taken over and just won't allow them to play. How many young wives get insufficient loving from their husbands because of his impotence? There are countless examples before our very eyes and it becomes even more heart breaking to know that we are the ones most responsible for our own situations. A shift towards more healthy options could work miracles for so many ailments. Give it a try. Try eating more nutritious foods for at least one or two months and see what happens. How do you feel? Be true to yourself!

Eating and drinking leafy green vegetables like spinach, fruits like sweet sop, and other natural wholesome foods like nuts and whole grains, help our bodies rejuvenate. Know that the human body is one of he most amazing mechanisms ever created. Know that we were born to live, and we are built to live long and strong lives. Our cells replenish themselves in the presence of oxygen. No cancer cell can develop and flourish in an oxygenated environment. Ask your doctor? Pure blood transports the best quality nutrients and the healthiest messages to our brains and to every other organ in the body. The purer the blood, the healthier the organs operate. The body in this case can be compared to the engine of a brand new vehicle. Everything runs smoothly.

Eating naturally as Mother Nature prescribed, maintains our balance with nature herself. When we eat the nuts, fruits, beans, berries, grains, and vegetables; and feast on green herbs, our cells identify with the natural formulas that make up these natural resources. Correct foods grow healthy and happy cells. Our cells do well because we are receiving life giving nutrients from these natural foods. A healthy cell is an energetic cell. Healthy cells promote healthy organs working in great condition. Healthy organs give power to healthy and energetic human bodies who are free to live full lives; as joyful as we choose to be. As long as the cells within our organs are receiving the correct amount of oxygen and other necessary nutrients, good health is certain. We remain free from impurities and we are sure to be happy and healthy. We should definitely strive to listen, learn to understand the human body, and support it fully with proper nutrients. Health is what really does a body good.

On the contrary, the results are totally opposite as with this unfortunate SAD (Standard American Diet) that the world has now adopted. This SADness is claiming so many lives and livelihoods that we really need to do some-thing about this situation NOW! When we reject the treas-ures that Mother Nature has provided and feast instead on artificial and chemical junk, we have basically signed our own death warrant – willingly. The build up of bad choles-terol, which is one of the main causes of poor circulation and heart conditions (cardio vascular diseases), has been directly linked to the overconsumption of fats, dairy prod-ucts and lack of exercise.

Junk foods like hamburgers and dairy products are loaded with salt, unsaturated fats, and unnatural sugars and don't do us any good either. These dangerous substances clog the veins and arteries creating a pressure and strain within our systems. The heart has to work that much harder to now pump the blood through our bodies. What comes next? Did I hear high blood pressure, strokes, heart attacks? It truly pays to understand how things happen. We should do our best to avoid foods that are not natural. The terrible byproducts of junk food are really what these germs and bacteria come to feast on. The more infested your cells become; the more likely you are to suffer from diseases.

Some animal flesh and fats take days and even weeks to be partially digested into the body. Some of us eat meat everyday; sometimes even twice and three times a day. Can you begin to understand what is happening inside of you? Hidden in dairy products are emulsifiers and other chemicals that cancer cells feed on. Look at it this way. There is a battle going on within you. The choice is yours as to who wins. Nature comes with cell wisdom. Life and health are her right and left hands. Processed foods come with chemical substances. Debt and hell are his right and left hands. Make the correct choice.

Every SAD meal increases our pain. The space within the veins and arteries become smaller and smaller. Clogged up veins and arteries will eventually lead to high blood pressure, strokes, and heart attacks etc. Along this road to debt/death, there are many signs. Regular visits at the hospitals and doctor's offices become more frequent. You begin to suffer from lack of energy, obesity, diabetes, shortness of breathe, poor circulation, cramps, aches and pains (whichever one comes first). It is now a proven fact that the SAD coupled with lack of exercise, is almost single handedly responsible for the current outbreak of CNCDs (Chronic Non-Communicable Diseases). These artificial foods are causing havoc throughout the nations of the world and everywhere its influence has spread. What should we do about it?

To rewire our circuits would be to reeducate ourselves. We should look at the food choices we make carefully, and choose those which add joy, health and laughter to our lives. We are natural beings and as such we should feed from nature's harvest. The choice is ours to make and it is never too late when we act now. Where there is enough will power, self determination opens up so many doors to victory that you may surprise yourself. Like Jimmy Cliff sang, *'you can get it if you really want. You can get it if you really want. But you must try...'* So try. Taste and see that Mother Nature is so very good to us. She is still fulfilling her promises to keep us and protect us always.

Creating New Lives

We are destined to live in the world nature intended and this book, like all the other bold works before it, is part and parcel of the process of getting us there. The idea is to get to that point where we are able to ask ourselves a question. The only way we increase learning is to invite it. Ask and you shall receive. Questions bring answers. Research and find the answer that you search for. You may not always be comfortable with the answer but be true to yourself.

The only thing constant is change. Nature has provided us with everything necessary to live a happy and healthy life. It should not be so hard to walk the ways of nature. The variety of choices available is abundant. The best experience comes straight from the tree itself.

Think of a coconut. This is one of nature's true gems for mankind. The water is filtered through the long fibers and contains natural electrolytes. Similar to the battery water found in cars, coconut water is battery water for humans. The flesh of this nut is so rich in nutrients and minerals that to list all the properties would be another book in itself. The healing properties associated with this coconut are unlimited. Research this information for yourself. Don't just take my word for it. Search and you will find.

Then there are avocadoes, cherries, apricots, grapefruits and oranges; herbs of every flavor, variety, and purpose; cashews, almonds, peanuts and pistachios; sweet potatoes, dasheen, pumpkins, and cucumbers, etc. There are so many choices that I could go on all day. Children naturally love fruits and vegetables. We are the ones who teach them to like this and not to like that. We should teach them to love nature. Eat healing foods, be happy, and love life.

Let the Truth be told; for every disease there is a remedy growing somewhere in the rain forest or in grand ma's backyard garden. Herbal medicine has performed miracles. The use of herbs to cure diseases has achieved results that fascinate even the best of medical professionals. When some claim that certain diseases are incurable, herbs come in and work healing magic. Everything is possible as long as you allow yourself to believe and act on it. Education will surely add life to our experience. When you know the facts and nutritional value of foods, even the things that you thought were not so nice now taste exquisite.

Get yourself a good blender and start having fun with combinations of fruits. Learn about the powers contained in the banana and his brother plantain. Juice spinach, cucumbers with carrots and drink to life. The tops of the beet root, yes the green part of it, also contain vital nutrients. Blend some in there. Add some to your beans and your stews. Love nature and nature will love you double. String beans are friends of the diabetic. Learn how these foods can help to balance your sugar and maintain insulin levels. Bitter herbs taste 'bad' to the tongue, true. But the cleansing effect they have on the blood, and especially the liver and the kidneys (the filters of the body) are unbeatable.

Keep in mind that these foods carry with them no side effects. They simply provide the nutrients that we need to function with life giving energy. Anyone who is interested in living a long, healthy and productive life should educate his or herself. Learn and explore the opportunities of nature.

The words in this book go beyond the boundaries of color, class, race, religion, and gender. Everyone who has a heart and is alive this very minute can gain and forever benefit from the abundant love that nature has prepared for us. Why wait?

The next section will introduce cell rejuvenating and mouth watering recipes. These are recipes that are not too difficult to prepare. Make sure you get everything on your shopping list. Free your mind and enter the kitchen. Create with joy. You are about to increase the love and admiration that your loved ones have for you. Righteousness is making the Right Choices! Be food good to yourself and others at all times.

Like the great Bob Marley sang to us, *"Emancipate yourselves from mental slavery; none but ourselves can free our minds..."* This is a process we can control. The decisions we make on a daily basis truly affect our lives sooner or later. Therefore we owe it to ourselves and our loved ones to learn as much as possible. There are many methods and means available leading towards living a more naturally fulfilling and joy-full life. Correct foods inspire correct thinking. A sound mind grows a strong and healthy body. Correct Foods are the best medicine known to man. Take the challenge. Educate yourself and live.

Are you going to allow yourself to be tricked or are you going to take a stand towards life choices? Ask yourself this question. Are you eating yourself to death? If your answer is yes, there is still time to make a change for the positive. Start eating to your health and prosperity. One wise love!

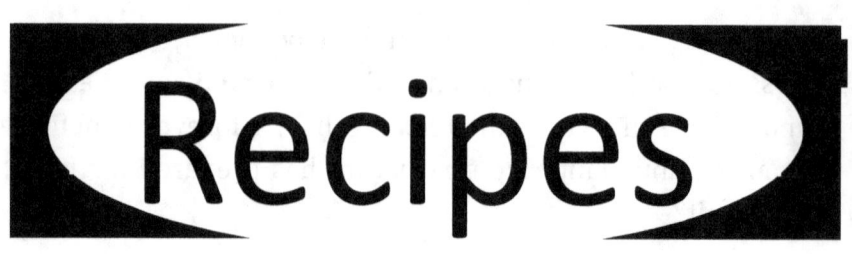

Recipes

The following pages contain recipes for a few healthy drinks, snacks, and natural meals that are sure to add to your health and wellness. You and your entire family will love the experience. Start looking at food from a brand new perspective. More over, Let your food be your medicine! Be wise. Eat and drink your way to Health, Joy, Achievement, and Prosperity.

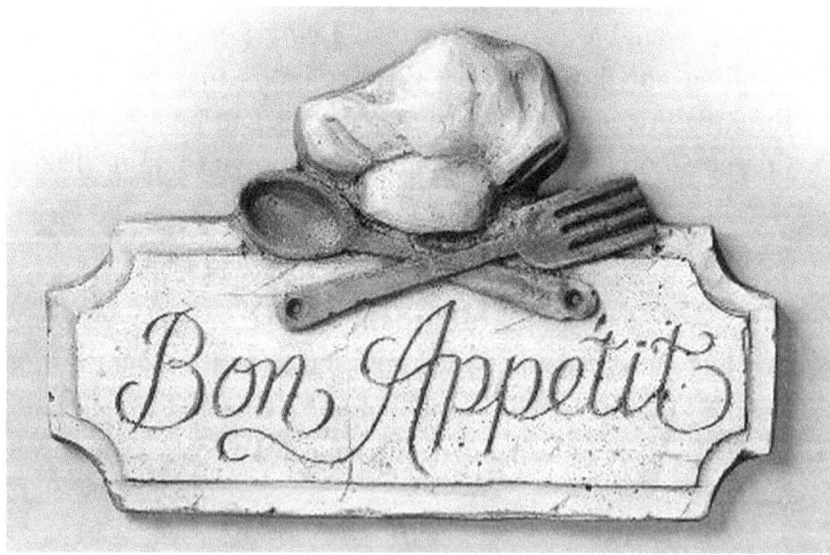

Chlorophyll Infusion

Ingredients:

A handful of spinach leaves

A handful of parsley leaves

1 stalk of celery

A handful of moringa leaves (optional)

two leaves of lettuce

raw ginger (to your desired strength)

honey/molasses/brown sugar to taste (optional)

Method of Preparation:

Wash all these lovely life giving greens thoroughly and place in a blender with a cup of spring clean water. Blend for about a minute. Repeat this process if you feel the need to. Pour content into a straining cloth or a strainer and squeeze out the goodness. This potent drink is a life giving elixir. Your cells will jump for joy and you will love it! Substitute other greens and make your own combinations.

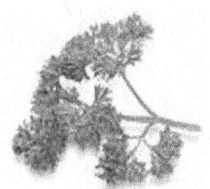 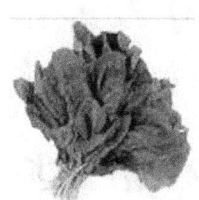

The Ultimate Smoothie

Ingredients:

1 small pineapple
1 ripe banana
1 small papaya
½ of a beet root
1 piece of raw ginger
2 tsb of honey/molasses (optional)
½ a cup of coconut milk or the soft flesh of the young coconut
1 cup of ice

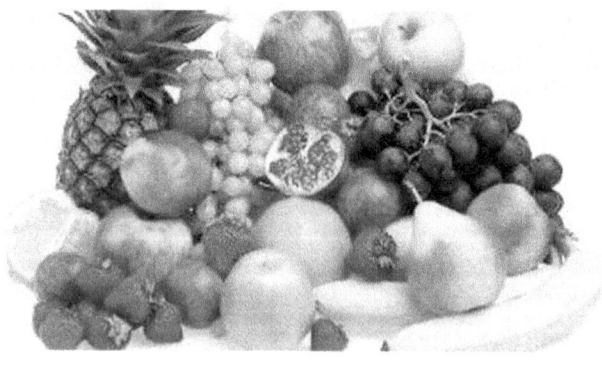

Method of preparation:

Peel pineapple carefully making sure that you remove the skin properly. Cut and slice into a bowl. Wash, slice open, and peel papaya. Remove the seeds. Wash and cut beet root. Now you are ready. Place all ingredients into a power blender and blend for a minute. Have your glass in hand. Heaven is just a blend of fruits away.

Pumpkin Butter

Ingredients:

1/2 of an 8lb pumpkin
1 whole onion
2 sprigs of chive, celery, parsley
3 seasoning peppers
1 sweet pepper
3 cloves of garlic
3 tbs of coconut oil
¼ cup of coconut milk
Salt to taste

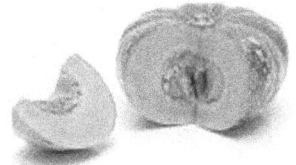

Method of Preparation:

Place a half a pot of water on the fire. Clean (remove the seeds), wash, and slice pumpkin (keep the skin; a lot of the nutrients are in there). Place into pot of bowling water and cover for about 10 to 15 minutes, or until pumpkin is soft enough to pierce though with a fork. Pour out hot water and let this cool for a few minutes. Place cooked pumpkin in a glass dish or bowl for crushing. Crush pumpkin thoroughly almost to a paste. Chop and cut up all seasonings, sweet pepper, garlic, and onions. Heat saucepan and when it is hot enough, add coconut oil and all the seasonings into the saucepan and let it simmer for about 2 minutes. Toss them around. Add the crushed pumpkin to the saucepan. Add coconut milk bit by bit while beating in the entire contents of the saucepan on a low fire. Keep whipping and adding the coconut milk until you have achieve a smooth consistency. Add salt to your taste. This could eventually replace your table or peanut butter. Spread on toast, sandwiches; top off rice or salad with this nutritious butter, use liberally. Store in glass jars and refrigerate for longer life. Add some rosemary if you plan to travel with it or send it to a friend.

Totally Vegan Pizza

Ingredients:

Pizza dough	Pizza topping
1lb whole wheat flour	1 slice of pumpkin (about 2lbs)
1 teaspoons of yeast	2 sprigs of chive, celery, parsley
1 teaspoons of salt	3 tomatoes
½ cup of corn meal	2 onions
¼ cup of Coconut Oil	1 head of garlic
½ cup of warm water	2 medium sized okras
	2 seasoning peppers
	1 bell pepper
	¼ cup of coconut milk
	2 tbs coconut oil
	salt to taste

Method of preparation:

Place whole wheat flour, yeast, salt, and cornmeal into a bowl and mix all these dry ingredients together. Add the coconut oil and mix in. Add warm water slowly bit by bit and knead thoroughly until the ball of dough does not stick to your fingers. Cover this dough and let it rise for at least 40 minutes.

In the mean time, clean and wash pumpkin, (I like to leave the skin on there) then grate into a bowl using the diamond side of the grater. Chop seasonings; slice the onion and bell pepper evenly from the top forming small and large circles. Place saucepan on a medium fire and when it gets hot enough add the coconut oil, some freshly grated garlic, and a dash of the coconut milk into the saucepan.

Add the pumpkin. After about 5 minutes or so add all the green seasoning including the okra into the saucepan and mix into the pumpkin. Add some coconut milk bit by bit and let this mixture stew down until the pumpkin melts down to a smooth spread. At this time add some more garlic and some of the sliced tomato. Turn off the fire and allow this to cool. Your dough should be ready by now. Preheat your oven to a temperature of about 300 degrees.

Place dough on a large enough rolling board or your counter top if is clean and large enough, and use a rolling pin (or a clean bottle) to roll out the dough evenly to the height of about 1/8 to 1/2 of an inch. Place crust on a pizza pan. Use a docker or a fork and form as many sink holes as possible (do not pierce through the crust). Slice tomatoes and spread evenly over the dough. You may sprinkle some fresh garlic strips and a pinch of salt if you wish on this tomato bed. Spread the pumpkin stew evenly over the tomatoes and design the top with the remaining slices of tomatoes, bell peppers, and onions in a creative design. Place pizza pan into the oven. Your pizza should be ready within 15-20 minutes. Once pizza is ready, remove from pizza pan, place unto the cutting board and slice accordingly with a pizza cutter or a sharp knife. Be careful ok. Pizza should be able to feed 7-8 people easily. Try different toppings!

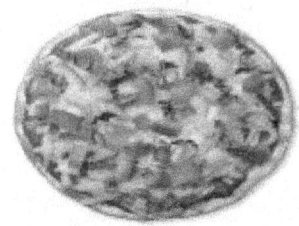

Broccoli Pockets

Ingredients:

Pastry
2lbs of whole wheat flour
½ cup of corn meal
1 tea spoon of yeast
¼ cup of coconut oil
1 tbs of vegetable shortening (optional)
1 tea spoon of salt
1 cup of warm water

Filling
1 package of broccoli
2 large tomatoes
1 large onion
1 bell pepper
1 medium sized carrot
2 sprigs of celery, parsley, chive
3 cloves of garlic
1 tsp of turmeric powder
2 tbs of coconut oil
½ cup of coconut milk (opt.)
Salt to your desired taste

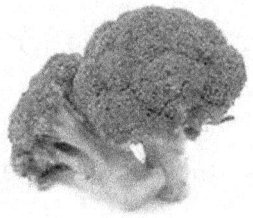

Method of Preparation:

(For pastry) in a large bowl, mix all dry ingredients (the flour, the corn meal, the yeast, and the salt) together. Add the coconut oil and vegetable shortening and mix properly into the flour mix. Add water slowly mixing thoroughly until the dough does not stick to your hand. Leave to rise for about thirty (30) minutes.

(For Filling) Chop onion, bell peppers, and fresh seasoning. Dice carrots into small cubes. Wash Broccoli and cut into chunks. (I like to bite into these juicy greens. You may like them smaller. Either way they taste delicious.) Grate the garlic and chop the tomatoes into reasonable sized chunks as well. Heat up saucepan for a minute on a medi-

um fire. Add some coconut oil to start. Add onions, half of the grated garlic, the Broccoli, some of the fresh green seasoning, and some coconut milk (or water). Allow to simmer for about five minutes. Add the tomatoes, bell pepper, the remainder of the fresh seasoning and garlic, the turmeric, and the carrots. Add some more milk or water to avoid sticking and to achieve a workable consistency. Let this simmer for an additional four to five minutes, stirring occasionally. Add salt to desired taste. Shut off.

Mix in dough once again. Make small dough balls, about the size of a medium lime or a golf ball. Allow to sit for about five additional minutes. Then with a rolling pin or a clean glass bottle, roll out dough balls onto a rolling board until flat and spread out. (One at a time please.) Place a spoonful of the Broccoli mix onto the center of the rolled out dough. Be sure you do not overload. Carefully take the top of the dough and place onto the opposite end as to seal, enclosing the Broccoli mix. Squeeze in the pocket with your fingers and seal pocket with a fork.

Be careful not to go too close as to puncture the pocket. Cut off the excess dough with a knife, leaving an inch or so of lip. Place on a floured baking pan. Repeat process for as many dough balls or mix that you have. Remember to preheat the oven at about 300 degrees. Place loaded baking pan into the oven and bake these goodies for about 10 minutes (or until bottom surface is golden brown). Make sure they don't stick to the pan. Flip pockets so the opposite side could receive this same golden brown treatment for about 5 to 7 minutes. Your family and friends will love you much more after this.

Vegan Banana Cheese

Ingredients:

1 hand of green banana
3 white potatoes
1 large onion
5 seasoning peppers
1 head of garlic
1 tsp turmeric
1 piece of raw Ginger
½ cup of coconut milk
2 sprigs of chive, celery, parsley
2 tbs of oil (coconut/olive/palm)
Salt to taste

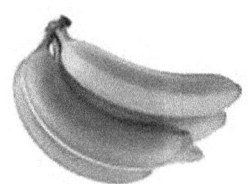

Method of Preparation:

Peel bananas and place in some salt water. Wash/scrub clean the potatoes (do not peel). On the small diamond side of the grater, grate the bananas. On the bigger diamond side of the grater, grate the potatoes. Heat pan, and place oil, a pinch of salt, and ¼ cp of coconut milk; then add the ginger, turmeric, some garlic, onion, and seasoning pepper. Allow to simmer for two minutes then add the grated banana and potato, and some more coconut milk (the coconut milk gives that cream cheese unique taste). Stew mixture for about 7-10 minutes, on a medium fire stirring occasionally to avoid sticking. Add green seasonings, and the balance of the onions and garlic. Use the remainder of the coconut milk to achieve the desired consistency. Add salt to your taste. This Vegan cheese can be used as a topping or served with green plantain or banana chips, toasted wheat slices, etc.

Coconut Doughnuts

This doughnut recipe is also a great base recipe, since other fruits and vegetable ingredients can be incorporated such as pineapple, apricots, carrots, beets, etc., to create incredible mouth watering combinations. This is not for everyday. But you can have some fun every now and again. Your children may have a different idea so be prepared.

Ingredients:

1 coconut   (blend coconut with just enough water for a smooth blend. The richer and creamier the milk, the more tasty these beauties will be)

2lbs of whole wheat flour

1tsp of yeast

1 ½ cups of sugar   (if you have some other natural sweetener like honey or Agave`, you may cut down on the amount of sugar)

¼ cup of coconut oil (palm or olive oil can work as well)

1L of palm/coconut oil (for frying)

½ tsp of cinnamon

A pinch of fresh ginger

Method of Preparation:

Mix all dry ingredients in a large mixing bowl. Add the ¼ of Coconut Oil and work into the mix. To avoid doughnuts getting too brown too fast, it is best to place the milk on a low fire and add and mix in the sugar making condensed milk. Add enough sweetened milk into the dry mix to form a smooth ball of dough that doesn't stick too much on your hands. Allow to sit and proof for at least 30 minutes.

Knead dough again and allow to sit for an additional 5 to 10 minutes. Then create balls of dough about the size of golf balls. Place oil in frying pan or deep fryer and heat on a medium fire. Ensure that oil is really hot (but not burning) before putting in the doughnuts. Place balls on rolling pan (sprinkle with flour) and roll out with a rolling pin to about an ½ inch. With a cutter, or the clean cover of a ginger wine bottle, make the whole in the center. Place into the frying pan or deep fryer and turn after one minute to avoid holes on the opposite side. Frying time for each should be about five to seven minutes.

(Suggested Toppings:

Chocolate fudge, shredded coconut, pineapples, glaze and flax/sesame seeds, nuts, honey, orange/lime/grapefruit glaze.)

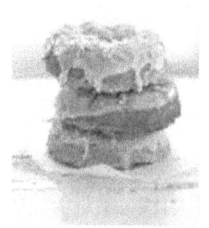

Provision Pie

This recipe will help all who taste this to discover a new reason to eat ground provisions. It doesn't always have to be the usual cook and chop into a plate. For this one we will be using Yams. However, you could use Dasheen, Tania, Green Banana, Green Plantain, even Sweet Potato; or a combination.

Ingredients:

2 yams (medium Size) or other ground provisions
½ cup of coconut milk
1 large onion
1 head of garlic
2 sprigs of chive/celery/parsley
4 seasoning peppers
1 bell pepper
1 tsp turmeric powder
2 carrots
2 large tomatoes
2 tsp coconut oil (optional)
salt to taste

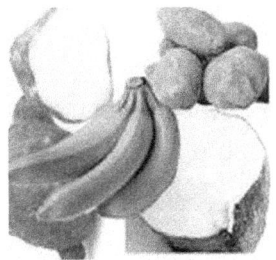

Method of Preparation:

Peel and wash provision. Cut in pieces and place in pot of boiling water with a pinch of salt for about 20 minutes or until soft enough for a fork to pierce through it easily. Remove from fire, drain, and allow to cool. In between time chop, onions, celery, parsley, chive and seasoning peppers.

Place a saucepan on medium heat with a ¼ of the coconut milk. Grate carrots, dice tomatoes, and place into pan with most of the onions, garlic, peppers, seasonings, and turmeric powder. Allow to simmer down on low heat for about ten minutes.

By this time the provision should now be easy to handle. Crush provision with a potato crusher or a fork as fine and smooth as possible. Add remainder of seasonings, salt to taste, and enough coconut milk to achieve the desired consistency.

Preheat oven to 300 degrees. Prepare baking dish by oiling it then add some flour to prevent sticking. Place half of the mixture and level into the baking dish. Place carrot and tomato stew onto the yams in the dish and level. Place remaining half of the mix onto the layer carrots and tomatoes and level nicely. Place baking dish into oven and bake for about 30 minutes or until the edges are golden brown.

Another option would be to add mixture of provision and vegetable mix together. Enhance taste if you choose to (extra onions, pepper sauce, etc.). Place in dish and press to shape. Let cool, cut and serve. No baking necessary for this one.

It is possible to have such exciting adventures with food. Your entire family will enjoy this; even those who claim that they do not like provisions and vegetables.

Carrot / Ginger Cake

Ingredients:

- 5 medium sized carrots
- 2 lbs of whole wheat flour
- 1 ½ cups of brown sugar
- 1 cup of coconut oil (palm/olive can be used also)
- 2 tsp of baking powder
- 1 tsp of cinnamon
- ¼ lbs of fresh ginger
- 1 tsp of egg replacer (optional)
- 2 cups of water (or orange juice)/ or half water half, orange juice

Method of Preparation:

Wash Carrots and chop into a powerful blender; (I use a Warin Pro, so make sure that yours is up to the task). Add sugar, oil, water, ginger, and cinnamon into the blender and blend for about 2 minutes or until contents are smooth (avoid clumps and grains). Put blended mix into a mixing bowl and add flour, baking powder, and egg replacer. Mix thoroughly with a cake mixer for about 4 to 5 minutes. (If you are like I am and don't have a cake mixer at all times, use a wooden spoon and beat the mix until smooth. This process usually takes 7 to 10 minutes and requires a bit of muscle).

Preheat oven to 350 degrees. Oil and flour baking pan. Add mixture and level out properly (make sure not to leave or create any air pockets). Bake for about 40 to 50 minutes at 300 degrees. Try adding some pineapple to this recipe. Your children and their classmates will soon be making orders!

Power Shake

Ingredients:

1 ripe banana
½ of an avocado
¼ cup of oats
2 tsp of flax seeds
2 cups of coconut milk
1 sprig of moringa (optional)
honey/molasses to taste (optional)
1 tsp of coconut/olive oil (option to really add some extra vigor to this)
1 cup of Ice

Method of Preparation:

Place all ingredients into a power blender and blend for about a minute.

This great shake could be enjoyed for breakfast, lunch, or dinner. Make your own combinations. Check your local farmers market for available fruits and vegetables. Or better yet, what do you have growing in your garden?

Bread Nut Ice Cream
(Non Dairy)

Ingredients:

1 lb of breadnut (cooked)
1 cup of coconut milk
2 tsp of cinnamon
½ a cup of toloma (arrowroot)
1 cup of brown sugar (add honey or molasses to use less sugar)

Method of Preparation:

Peel Breadnut. To 1 cup of boiling water add toloma. Mix until smooth and allow to cool to room temperature. Add arrowroot (cooled) and all other ingredients into the power blender and blend for 2 minutes. Empty the contents into ice-cream bowl. Place in the freezer for ½ an hour. Remove container from freezer and once again blend for an additional 2 minutes. Empty contents in a bowl and freeze until set and ready. You will soon realize that Breadnut is one of nature's best kept heavenly secrets; abundantly found on the nature isle of Dominica. Come to Natural Livity Vegan Café`, email or call us. We will be happy to introduce you to some of these recipes and so much more.

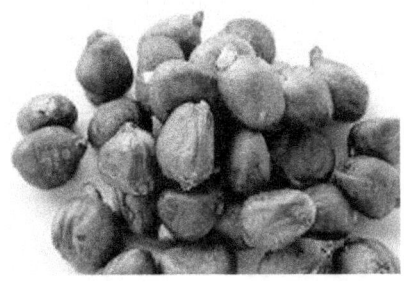

About the author:

Jaimie "Dr. J" Cornelius is th e founder of Natural Livity Inc.; a personal Health care service provider primarily focused on using natural foods and education to achieve nutritional balance and holistic healing.

Natural Livity Inc. has been in operation for the past eleven (11) years and our services have grown to include Catering (Vegan Food), Consultations and Cooking Classes, Seminars, Eco Tours and Retreats, and Entertainment {Live Music and Artists} Packages. Our treatments focus on correcting stress, fatigue, obesity, diabetes, cardio vascular complications, cancers, and other forms of Chronic Non Communicable Diseases or CNDCs as they are commonly called. We help you find the peace of mind, joy and happiness that you rightfully deserve.

He is also very happy to have been one of the nine (9) founding directors who initiated the formation of an amazing organization, the Dominica Spa Health and Wellness Association or DSHWA. We see this organization as a vehicle designed to drive Dominica up the road to attaining its rightful position as the premier health and wellness destination of the world. We look forward to welcoming you to this beautiful island experience and catering to your every need.

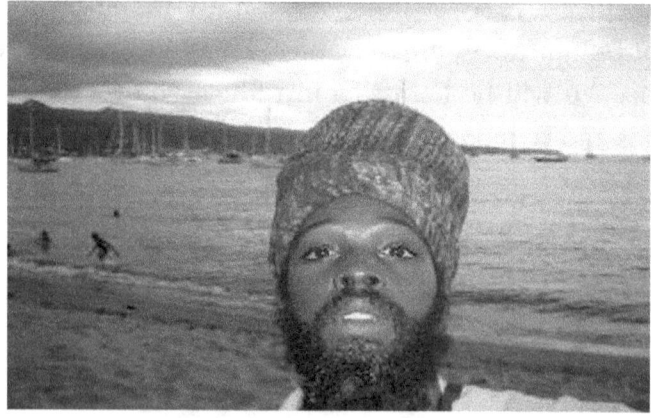

Editor: Mrs. Jane Cornelius
Cover Design ©: Francis Destouche
Computer Graphic Design © : Pops Morris